I0436875

Real Solutions To Children's Health

by
Anne Arsenault

Bloomington, IN 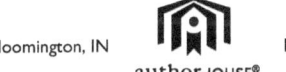 Milton Keynes, UK

AuthorHouse™
1663 Liberty Drive, Suite 200
Bloomington, IN 47403
www.authorhouse.com
Phone: 1-800-839-8640

AuthorHouse™ UK Ltd.
500 Avebury Boulevard
Central Milton Keynes, MK9 2BE
www.authorhouse.co.uk
Phone: 08001974150

All rights reserved. No part of this book may be reproduced or transmitted by any means or in any form, mechanical or electronic, or electronically processed, photographed, recorded in audio form, photocopied for public or private use nor stored in a retrieval and/or information storage system, in any form without the prior written permission of the publisher and/or the copyright holder, or by any means without permissionin writing from the author, Anne Arsenault.

© 2006 Anne Arsenault. All rights reserved.

First published by AuthorHouse 11/30/2006

ISBN: 978-1-4259-7630-9 (sc)

Printed in the United States of America
Bloomington, Indiana

This book is printed on acid-free paper.

Disclaimer: The information in this book is based on published and unpublished sources and it is the opinion of the author. The author has made every attempt to provide accurate information, but every child and situation is unique. The purpose is for educational and research purposed only and should not be construed as giving medical advice. The author of this book neither prescribes any technique, nor dispenses medical advice as a form of treatment for medical problems without the direct or indirect advice of a physician. If the reader uses the information to solve their health problems, they are prescribing for themselves in which case they are exercising their constitutional right, but the author and publisher assume no responsibility for their actions.

Make sure you visit your doctor as needed and go to emergency if the condition is serious.

To contact the author go to: amal153@yahoo.ca
www.healthbrights.com
www.childhealthebook.com

Cover Photos by James MacMullen
www.jemshots.com

digitaldirect@mac.com

TESTIMONIALS

"There is so much information in this book, it's almost too much"!

R Bruce Banman Doctor of Chiropractic

"You have done a marvelous job explaining in easy to understand terms for children and their parents how important it is to have a good diet and how to avoid **junk food** (mostly processed food with **MSG** and other chemical food additives) and dangerous pop drinks with **Aspartame**.

Remember: **YOU ARE WHAT YOU EAT!**

"If we don't take care of our children who are our future, we will have no future!"

Yours in health,

Klaus Ferlow, President & founder of FERLOW BOTANICALS, Div. of Ferlow Brothers Ltd, Vancouver, B.C., www.ferlowbotanicals.com

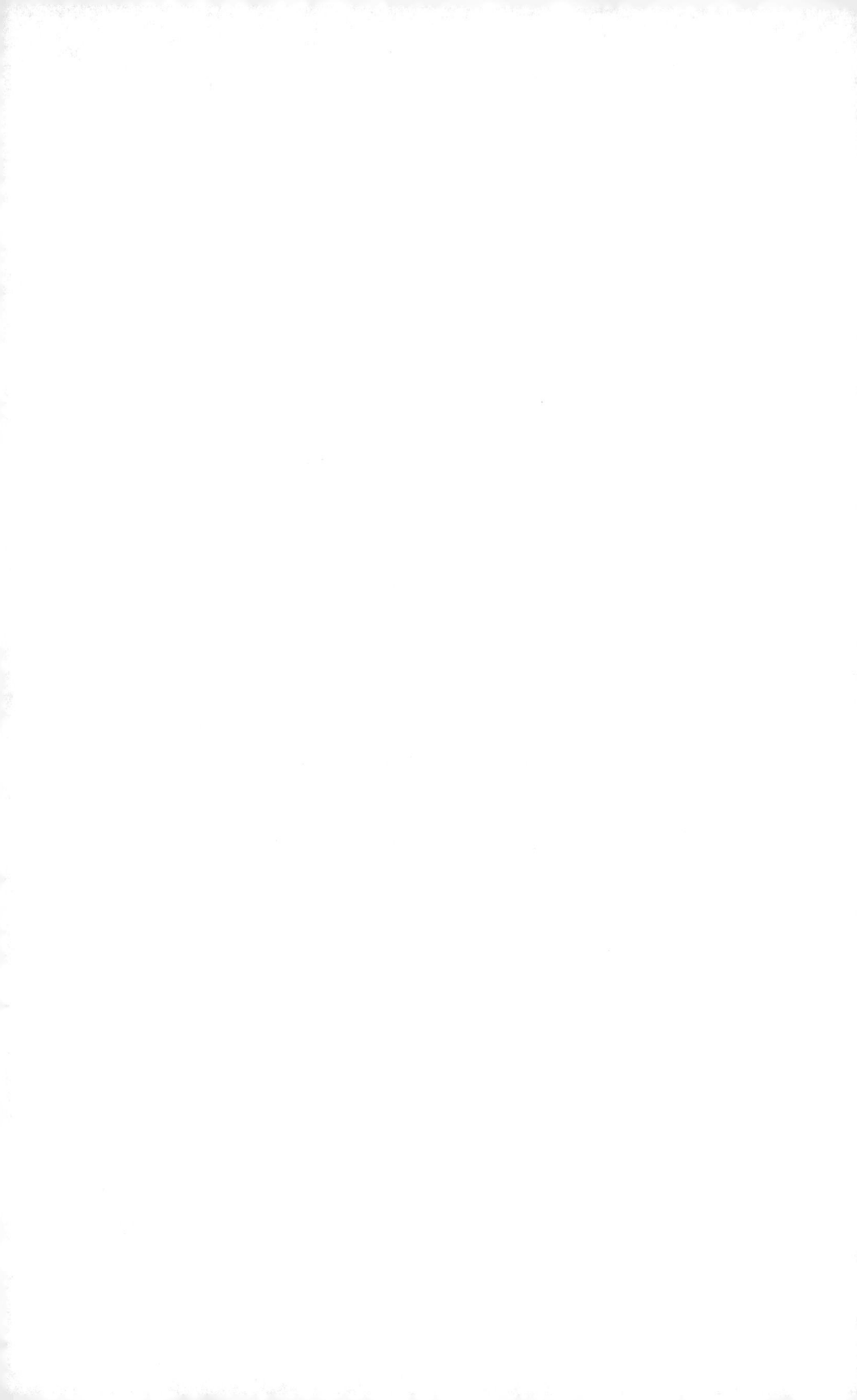

DEDICATION

I would like to thank my Mother and my Oma, for bringing me up in a healthier home. I would also like to thank my family and my wonderful friends for all the love, support and for believing in me. Last, but not least, my daughter for her unconditional love.

TABLE OF CONTENTS

INTRODUCTION

Our children are our future so we need to teach them health. They say the best way to teach is by example. Learning to live a healthy lifestyle is teaching your children what it takes to live healthy. It is our responsibility to teach them health.

What they eat and drink can make a big difference in their behaviour. Children can have less mood swings and be calmer and less out of control. Most times it is as simple as taking them off artificial colourings (red) and cutting back on the sugar. Other times you need to get them allergy tested or take them off of things like dairy, wheat, chocolate, corn or whatever else tests positive. Diet plays a much larger role in health and behaviour than we realize.

Supplements can also make a difference, but knowing what to give, how much, and in the right forms, can be a challenge. Certain conditions give us signs that the body is lacking specific vitamins and minerals. Herbs can be taken to boost the immune system, strengthen the respiratory system, and for many other uses. You just need to lower the dose according to weight and age.

Health is a lifestyle. You will not get healthy by just changing one thing, but each thing you do change will be another step towards your goal of health. To provide a positive atmosphere that will nurture and teach your child to become an independent, responsible member of society is the parent's goal. Let the child become what they desire yet still set up proper structure. Keep the communication lines open and teach them consequences, especially when they choose not listen to us. Teach them love and respect for themselves, for others, animals, and the world around them. Parenting uses all our resources, our creativity, our patience and much more, but the experience of watching your child grow, develop, and then make their way in society compares to nothing else.

PART ONE

CHAPTER ONE
WATER, JUICE and OTHER FLUIDS

After oxygen, water is the most needed substance. It makes up more than 60% of our body weight. Children have a greater risk of dehydration, especially when there is a fever, diarrhea, vomiting or hot temperatures. It takes only a 10% loss of your body's water to create fatigue, mental confusion and problems with the body's temperature regulation. If someone cannot handle the summer heat, try giving him or her more water.

Water is used in many important ways in the body: temperature regulation, regular bowel functioning, chemical reactions, transport for vitamins and minerals, and for the organs to stay lubricated and absorb shock.

An adult should have eight cups of purified water a day. Divide that in half for children half the size and in half again for smaller children. If your child will not drink this amount, then try some of the following suggestions.

· watered-down natural juice
· a water bottle
· hot/warm water
· Herbal tea (no caffeine)

- ice water
- a squeeze of lemon/lime
- the "Cheers" game
- your example of drinking more
- eating more raw fruits and vegetables.

Playing "Cheers" is when you clink glasses together, then both have a drink. Please remember to never force them to drink water as this will cause them to rebel and drink less.

Juice is really not a needed item in our diet. Many of the juices on the market are full of sugar, artificial colours and flavours—there is not much real juice in them! When you do give juice, give only natural (100%) juice and water it down—a glass or two a day, not all day. The reason juice, even natural juice, is not healthy is that it contains the sugars from the fruit and not the fiber. When you eat the whole fruit, the fiber slows the release of the sugar into the bloodstream. Pop, Kool-Aid and other drinks like them contain artificial colours and flavours, along with either sugar or aspartame. Artificial colours, especially red, have been known to increase hyperactivity and other behaviour problems in children. Aspartame has been documented to set off seizures in children that had no previous history of seizures. Colas are not for children.

Let's talk about soda pop. Soda pop is one of the main items that are causing obesity and sickness in out children. Each can contains many teaspoons of sugar, high fructose corn syrup (a sugar), artificial colours and flavours and often caffeine and/or aspartame. One can, can contain 12 teaspoons of sugar; this amount of sugar will shut down your immune system for hours, which means your body will not be able to fight any virus you come in contact with. The high fructose corn syrup is being linked to childhood obesity. The amount of calories in one pop, 800 calories for one Big Gulp, also leads to obesity. Of course, our children don't need more artificial colours and flavours. The caffeine is highly addictive and will cause withdrawal symptoms in your child. Do you really want your child being addicted to such a drug? Aspartame, the artificial sweetener, has been known to cause seizures in children that never had them previously and it also causes more cravings for sweets. Drinking pop has been linked with these conditions: ADD, Insomnia, Kidney stones, Osteoporosis, Tooth decay and Obesity.

Dairy products will be discussed in another chapter so I will only say that if you know or suspect your child is reacting to milk then choose the alternatives of Soy, Goat, or Rice milks. There are also good Soy formulas on the market now.

Ice cream can either be natural or chemical made. The regular ice cream is just milk by-products with chemicals added for colours and flavours, so make sure you read the ingredients!

Remember that after oxygen, water is the most abundant substance in the body and needs to be replenished daily. Thirst is the last sign that the body is dehydrated so include lots of fresh fruits, vegetables, and water in your child's diet.

CHAPTER TWO
HOW TO FEED YOUR CHILDREN

How and what you feed your child, even at an early age, can make a much bigger influence on their life than you think. If you feed them processed, sugary, refined foods, they soon develop taste buds only for those foods. As they grow up eating their diet of predominately processed food, diabetes, cancers, heart disease, behaviour problems and other conditions begin to develop. Studies show that signs of heart disease are seen in children as young as three-years-old. Combine this diet with lack of exercise and we really have a problem. If the pattern is not broken, they will feed their children the same way and so on through the generations.

Babies do not need sugar and salt so read the ingredients or make your own baby food. You can purée cooked vegetables or fruits and then freeze them in ice cube trays. Defrost as many as you need for the meal. Do not heat up the food in a microwave as your baby can easily get burned this way. Remember to give them whole fruit, not just the fruit juice.

Toddlers should be fed **vegetables**. If they don't like a certain vegetable, try others. Be creative if you need to—cut them into different shapes, put them in soups, and provide dips. Always be the example and eat them yourself. If you cannot grow your own organic garden, buy as much organic as you can; BC Hot House products use very little, in any, chemical pesticides. If you cannot get fresh, frozen vegetables are the next best thing. I always keep frozen peas and other vegetables in the freezer. It makes a quick snack or combined with brown rice, a healthy dinner. Cook the brown rice in a natural, MSG-free soup cube for more flavour. If you choose to feed meat, combine it with non-starchy vegetables.

Fruits are also important. 70% of our diet should be fruits and vegetables. Fruits should be eaten alone. Fruits have a shorter digestion time and can cause gas if eaten with meats which have a much longer digestion time. Eat fruit for breakfast or for snacks. Remember that children can easily choke on fruits such as whole grapes. Dried fruits also make a good snack to carry with you. You can even dehydrate apples at home, but only give a small amount as they will swell in the stomach. Raisins are best organic, as grapes are high in pesticides. They are a good source of iron, too.

If you are still having a problem feeding them fruits and vegetables, try a Rebar. It has two cups of fruits and two of vegetables in each bar, yet doesn't taste like vegetables. Even just a piece of the Rebar is good. Also Juice+ Gummies contain 17 fruits, grains and vegetables, in a tasty gummy form. A serving of vegetables to a toddler is a lot smaller than for adults so give them a smaller portion. Try taking them out for Chinese food. Chop Suey contains lots of vegetables—request no MSG when ordering. Their taste buds will change with time and day to day. A vegetable they didn't like might now become their favorite and vice versa. There are also things like Phytobears on the market, which contain fruits and vegetables in a gummy bear.

Whole Grains are also an important part of our diet. There are many sprouted whole grain breads on the market now, so get them used to the taste of the grains and away from white bread. Brown rice is a great food, rich in B vitamins and minerals. Breakfast cereals should be whole grain. There are many great companies such as: Nature's Path, Lifestream, Barbara's, Erewhon and Kashi. Pasta can also be made from whole grains—you can get pasta made from brown rice, whole wheat, Kamut, Spelt and multi-grains. Any white flour product turns into sugar in the bloodstream so keep it to a minimum. You can use whole wheat in your baking, just remember that it is a little heavier and might make the product a bit dryer. Whole wheat pastry flour is also available. The fiber in the whole grain is needed to help clean the colon and to slow the release of sugar into the bloodstream. There are also a lot more vitamins and minerals in whole grains than in the refined flours.

Protein is also required in a healthy diet. There are many different forms of protein: meat, fish, dairy, beans, peas, nuts, seeds, soy, whole grains, and protein powders. Make sure your child gets some protein every day. If a child does not want to eat meat, do not force them, just find other proteins. Dairy contains protein, but what if your child is dairy intolerant? Goat and Soya now come in a wide range of products. Besides milk, you can get cheeses, yogurt, and even ice cream. Try feeding your child beans and other legumes. You never know what they will like and there are many great recipes available now. Vegetables like peas and corn contain protein—peas and brown rice are a complete protein. Other grains like Kamut, Spelt, Quinoa, Millet and Amaranth are high in protein. Nuts and seeds are easily choked on when a child is small so use nut butters instead—almond, sesame (Tahini), soy, Mystery butter, cashew, along with peanut butter are only a few of the varieties on the market. Spread them onto toast, crackers, rice cakes, or use them in your baking. Another great way to get protein into your child's diet is to use protein powders—most stores carry Whey, Soy, and Rice. Make sure it is not a weight loss formula containing Thermogenic

Herbs, as these are usually not meant for children. Check for artificial sweeteners like Aspartame, as it has been known to set off seizures in children. We make a nice breakfast drink containing bananas, frozen strawberries (or other berries), soy milk, flax oil, greens and of course, protein powder.

Give your child a choice of a few fruits and a few vegetables. Research has shown that children will eat more fruits and vegetables this way. Less is more—by putting out only a few vegetables, they will eat more than if you put out lots. Remember, you can always give them more. Make sure you explain that a treat is a treat and not a regular part of the diet. Never feeding them treats is not the answer as when they are older they might choose to do the opposite and eat mostly treats. Moderation and education is the key. Never fight with your child about eating, just be firm, consistent and most of all, set an example.

Don't expect to change your diet overnight—everything takes time. Make small goals for yourselves, such as: this week we will drink this much water, next week we will eat brown rice three times, and the next week we will add these vegetables to our diet. After a while, it will become second nature for you to include more whole grains, fruits and vegetables in your diet. You will find that you and your family will be eating less junk food as your body gets filled with nutrition.

CHAPTER THREE
FATS

It is so important that we feed our children the right fats and oils. The body requires fat for protecting the organs, making the hormones, helping form every cell membrane and for the health of the immune and cardiovascular system. Your brain should be 40% fat. Your nerve endings require fat and it is also needed for the cell's energy production. These are just some of the uses of fats in the body; they play a very important role.

An expectant mother should consume these Essential Fatty Acids (EFAs) in order for the baby's brain to develop properly. When I was pregnant with my daughter, I craved walnuts. When I really looked at the walnut I realized it looks like a brain. I also took salmon and flax oils. During pregnancy do not take Borage or Evening Primrose Oil. Eating more fish is beneficial for the baby's brain.

As a society we have been taught to be scared of fat and it has led to a great deficiency. As each generation is born, we become more and more deficient. Fat is not bad. Eating the wrong fats and not eating the right fats is the problem. The EFAs must be consumed; the body cannot make them. If the mother is deficient, the child will be too. The child will develop conditions such as: cradle cap, eczema, dry skin and hair, allergies, immune problems, growth problems, vision and learning problems, behavioural disturbances and ADD (attention deficit disorder.) Lack of EFAs is not the only reason for these conditions, but these are some of the signs of an EFA deficiency.

When we crave fried foods and other junk foods high in fat we actually need the good fats. As you consume these essential fatty acids you will find the cravings for these junk fats will begin to diminish. As a parent, you should be the example by eating more good fat and don't worry, it won't cause you to get fat. The right fats help you to lose weight as they nourish and build the body. They must be cold pressed and in dark bottles as heat, light and oxygen turns them into trans fats (bad fats.) Do not cook with them! Consuming a variety like: extra virgin olive oil, flax oil, salmon oil, hemp oil, combinations (Udo's Oil, Essential Balance,) eating avocados, raw nuts and seeds is the way to go. If you must fry, do it with butter and coconut oil as they can be heated to a higher temperature. If you buy flax oil or its combination, freeze it, or use it within 6 weeks after it is opened. The oil does not freeze solid. An adult can also take the capsules but remember, it takes about nine capsules of flax oil to make 1 tablespoon of the oil (one tablespoon per 100 lbs)

A child can take the liquid oil or take supplements like Focus, Learning Factors, Efalex Focus, etc. These come in smaller capsules shaped like a little football. Take the dosage stated on the bottle according to size/age. These are specifically recommended for children with ADD, hyperactivity, learning disabilities and other behavioural problems. If you want to take the liquid oil, there are ways to disguise the taste. Mix it into a protein blender drink, make your own salad dressing, mix it into your butter, and pour a little on rice, pasta or hot cereal after it is cooked. Make sure they cannot taste it and in some cases, that they do not see you put it in! The dosage should be according to 1 tablespoon to 100 lbs, ½ for 50 lbs., and so on. When you make salad dressing, you can mix it with other cold pressed oils (canola, olive, sunflower, etc.,) lemon juice, apple cider vinegar and other spices. Do not cook with the butter that has the cold pressed oil in it. Butter is better than margarine, unless there is a problem with dairy. If you use margarine, just use the non-hydrogenated ones.

Studies have shown that with the right diet and supplements a child will calm down and begin learning again. After taking flax oil for the first time, I felt calmer and my neck pain began to subside. Along with water and a proper diet, it is also a great remedy for constipation, especially with children. EFAs help the body with so many things: anxiety, depression, pains in muscles and joints, skin, dandruff, neck and back pain, food allergies, fatigue, a feeling of calmness and the list goes on.

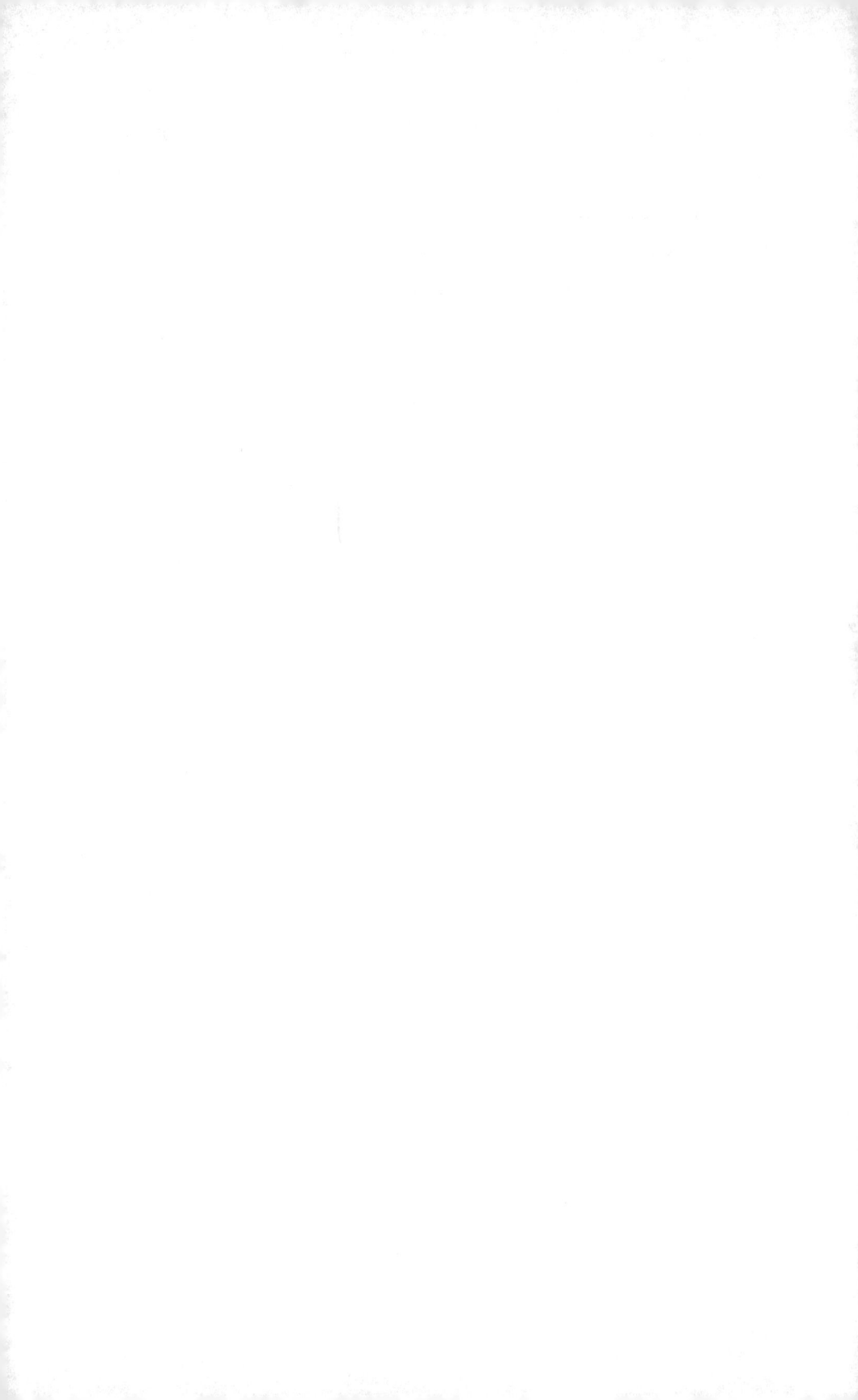

CHAPTER FOUR
DAIRY PRODUCTS

For years we have heard "milk does the body good," but the concept is not right for every child. Many children and also adults cannot digest milk—it causes discomfort such as: ear infections, rashes, colic, diarrhea, respiratory problems, eczema, hives, behaviour disturbances and other gastrointestinal problems. Milk is meant for baby cows and they grow up faster than human babies so it contains too much fat and too much protein for the human body. Although it does contain calcium, calcium needs the mineral magnesium to absorb properly and milk has little, if any, magnesium. More and more people are taking themselves and their children off of milk for these reasons and more.

The best dairy products to consume are the ones that have been fermented and contain friendly bacteria (acidophilus): yogurt, kefir, quark and other products like them. The proteins have been broken down and the fact that they contain acidophilus makes them more digestible. Make sure you read the ingredients in the yogurt as many contain fillers, artificial colours, flavours, sugars and even aspartame. The healthiest choice is the natural plain yogurt.

Organic dairy products are becoming more and more popular. Regular milk contains hormones, antibiotics and even pesticides. The cows are often not treated humanely. For these reasons, many consumers are turning to organic, especially for their children.

For those who do not react to dairy, it can be a source of protein, fat and B12. Blood type B's, seem to tolerate dairy the best. Often a child who craves milk is the one who is reacting to it, so pay attention to what your child is craving and any reactions they might be having. Keep a journal if you need to. Remember a good natural yogurt is often tolerated, even if milk is not.

Other conditions that are being linked to milk (dairy) consumption are: juvenile insulin-dependent diabetes[1], acne, digestive problems, certain cancers[2], allergies and a higher risk of hip fractures[3]. The study done on diabetes and milk consumption was published in the New England Journal of Medicine. Milk is not the only cause, as genetics and other dietary factors play a role. If you choose not to use dairy at all, there are many products on the market made from goat, soy and rice. You will find milks, yogurts, cheeses, ice creams and more made out of dairy alternatives. If your child will not eat plain yogurt, here are some ideas:

- put some in a blender drink
- make a vegetable dip
- combine it with fruit
- mix some natural fruit spread, or maple syrup into the yogurt.

Whether to consume dairy products or not, is totally your decision, but watch out for the warning signals of your child reacting to milk. Also remember to read the label and choose the natural dairy products.

CHAPTER FIVE
ALLERGIES, SENSITIVITIES

Allergies and sensitivities are a broad subject so we will only cover the basics in this chapter. More information can be found in Part Two of this book under "Allergies" and in the listing of more in-depth books at the back of the book.

These two conditions can affect every area of your body, including the brain. They can produce different symptoms at different times with the same allergen. Often what the child is reacting to is the very thing he/she craves. There are two ways of finding out the allergens—go to a Naturopath, or go to someone else who can test for these, and/or keep your own journal and do your own elimination diet. Buying a book on the subject is a must. Here are just a few of the symptoms:

- food cravings
- fatigue
- insomnia
- ear infections
- hives
- eczema
- rashes
- headaches

- stuffy nose
- ADD
- hyperactivity
- hypoglycemia
- depression
- asthma
- immune problems
- diarrhea
- constipation
- aching muscles
- bed-wetting
- colic
- digestive problems
- irritability
- fatigue upon waking
- dark or puffy eyes

As you can see, there are so many symptoms and some of them even contradict each other.

So, where do you start? First, look at your child's diet—read the labels and see what is really in the food you eat. Artificial colourings should be eliminated. Then check for things like MSG, aspartame and artificial flavourings. Milk, wheat, gluten, corn, and chocolate are the first things to remove in an elimination diet. You might have to go further with the wheat and eliminate all gluten products, wheat, oats, barley, rye and triticale. Always read the labels because many products which contain milk and wheat might not occur to you. These days there are so many more products made without the dairy, wheat, gluten and other allergens.

What causes these allergies? Genetics, eating the same foods every day, babies being fed formula, stress, misalignment of the spine, mercury fillings, lack of good bacteria in the gut, and being bombarded with chemicals in our food and environment. Our body becomes overloaded with chemicals foreign to the body and it becomes toxic. The chemicals used in and around the house are actually the most toxic. All the way from weed killers, to cleaners, sprays, shampoos, deodorants, perfumes and even our laundry soaps. All of these are toxic to our body. If a child has a skin or respiratory problem, take a look at the chemicals you use every day and change to natural ones. Here are some of the natural companies: Nature Clean, Seventh Generation, Ecover, Carina, Nature's Gate, Jason, Burt's Bees, Druide, Simply Clean, Kiss My Face, Desert Essence, and more.

What is an elimination diet? You eliminate the suspected food for a week to see if your symptoms go away. Then you eat it and wait for up to two days to see if the symptoms return. You can do this with each suspected food item. It is important to keep a daily journal of what is consumed—the symptoms and their times.

It will take time to figure things out, so be patient, one step at a time. Remember, it is often what is craved and eaten in large amounts, or daily, that is the allergen.

CHAPTER SIX
SUPPLEMENTS

What supplements should I give my child? There are so many supplements on the market now, but how do you know what your child needs and what is good quality? Some companies are in business to make natural, quality products and some are just in it for the money. Look for natural colours, flavours and no aspartame in the vitamin products. Companies like: Quest, Swiss, Natural Factors, Nulife, Albi, Sisu, Prairie Naturals, Now, Food Science and Bioforce make high quality product. Most, if not all, of these companies test the products on a regular basis; they test for impurities and that the ingredients are in the bottle in the said amount. Some of them even test to see if the multi-vitamin and calcium-magnesium actually absorb in a solution that is similar to the liquid in our stomachs. The best product will do nothing if it does not absorb into the body.

The first thing to look for in a **multi-vitamin-mineral pill** (chewable) is for no aspartame. Next, check for natural colours and flavours. Give your child the vitamin with breakfast or lunch. When your child does not eat enough fruits and vegetables, give them Juice+ Gummies for kids, they will provide the extra servings of fruits and vegetables they don't eat. If your child is experiencing growing pains, teeth grinding, or chocolate cravings, **calcium-magnesium** is a good choice. You can purchase this in chewable or liquid. Insomnia can be helped with calcium-magnesium; therefore, you can take it with a snack in the evening.

If you find your child's immune system is weak and he/she's catching a lot of colds and flues, there are ways to build it up. Cut back on the sugar and white flour products in their diet. Also cut back on the refined, hydrogenated fats. **Vitamin C** with bioflavonoids, come in many natural chewable tablets. For a child under two, you can get the Swiss 100mg, or break a 500mg up and eat the rest yourself. Over two, they are usually big enough for the 500mg a day. **Zinc lozenges** can be used as soon as they are old enough to suck on a lozenge. Check the strength of the zinc—usually 5-25mg per lozenge. For a toddler, get a lozenge that is 10mg and give a couple per day until the cold/cough is better. If a child is half the size/weight of an adult then give half the adult dose. If the child is a quarter the size, give them a quarter the adult dose. Just as you would not give hard candies to babies, do not give lozenges to babies. Always read the label and purchase products with natural colourings, flavourings and no aspartame.

Herbal medicine can be useful in building the immune system. Herbs like Echinacea, Astragalus and others can be bought in liquid form and added to a natural juice. Follow the directions on the bottle for children or use the directions in the last paragraph for the amount given. There are specific immune formulas on the market for children. Echinacea should only be given for a week or so, but can be given often throughout the day, every 2 hours. Water down the juice because too much juice will put down the immune system. There are some herbal cough syrups on the market geared toward children. Herbal ear drops are also useful, Master Formula and St. Francis Herbs are good ones. If your child will drink cooled herbal teas like, catnip, fennel, peppermint, ginger, licorice and chamomile, they will often soothe the tummy and calm the child. To really understand herbs, get yourself a good book.

Another way to treat your child's problems is by **homeopathy**. There are companies like Boiron, Hylands and Dolisos that make actual children's lines. You will find products for: teething, colic, sleeping, cold, flues, coughs, bedwetting, bruising, and more. **Bach Flower Remedies** work on specific emotional traits. Rescue Remedy is the most popular, used for calming after traumatic events. Follow the directions on the bottle on how to administer them. Homeopathy stimulates the body's natural defense mechanisms to help the body heal itself. Get a book on the single remedies or visit a homeopathic doctor to find remedies for more specific problems. These remedies are virtually non-toxic.

Another thing that can be used for children is **acidophilus**. For children you can get it in powder or a chewable tablet. A capsule can also be opened and poured into a natural yogurt. This should be given for the two weeks after antibiotics have been given. **Aromatherapy** is also good; certain scents can have a calming affect on the child. You can purchase them in specific formulas, or make your own. Always use a carrier oil, almond is good; do not put them directly on the skin. The mixture can be massaged into the skin, diffused into the air and put into the bath. Take care, as they are stronger than they appear; only a couple drops are usually needed.

There are so many products on the market geared towards children. Try the natural soaps, shampoos, and skin creams made for children. The chemicals we put on our skin also make their way into the body. Just remember to make sure the product is natural and read the appropriate dosages. If the condition is serious or you feel you need a professional diagnosis, take your child to a hospital, to your doctor, or to a clinic.

CHAPTER SEVEN
ALTERNATIVE THERAPIES

There are many alternative therapies available that can benefit your child. Touch has been shown to improve a child's development and growth. Chiropractic has been used, with good results. Aromatherapy and homeopathy are becoming more popular. Even acupuncture is being used for children now. If a child has been through traumatic events, then there are counseling and other therapies available. Art therapy is a good choice for a child. If your child has a lot of anger it is important to deal with this anger appropriately and to find the cause of it. There is always a reason, whether your child can put it into words or not. Children are very sensitive.

Massage can be a bonding time between parent and child. It should be done in a firm, slow manner to produce a soothing affect. There are also many other benefits to massage: it assists the lymphatic system in cleansing the body of toxins, relieves tension, improves sleep, helps for better growth in body and brain and increases self awareness and esteem. Never massage a premature baby without first asking a doctor. Dr. James Prescott[4] did a study in the 1980's which found that children that had been brought up with more touch were less likely to become violent than those brought up with little touch. There are classes, books and videos to teach you the techniques, or take your child to a registered massage therapist.

When a child is born, it is traumatic to the body, especially the spine. Chiropractic can help, even from a young age. Choose a chiropractor you are comfortable with, as there are different techniques available. Over the years of playing, sports, and falls, your child's spine can be put out of place (subluxation). By fixing the subluxation, the child can have better balance, stride, digestion, immune, posture, growth and over all better health. Conditions such as: allergies, asthma, colic, digestive problems, immunity and ear infections have shown improvement with chiropractic help. SIDS has been linked with a subluxation of the neck and also with smoking. It is much easier to fix a subluxation in a child than in an adult. When my daughter started running I could see her left foot was pointing out. I saw a great improvement in this after a couple treatments. After her very first treatment as a baby, she proceeded to empty her bowels for quite a while after the chiropractor had left the room. The chiropractor needs to only use a couple fingers with a baby. Waiting until you are older to go means that your muscles are set in the position of the subluxation and it will be more difficult for the adjustment to hold.

Aromatherapy is gaining in popularity and can be useful for children. Just follow these rules:

- No oils on babies under three months
- From 3-18 months use them cautiously
- 18 months to 5 years, double the amount of carrier oil.
- During pregnancy you must be careful as a lot of oils should not be used, consult a professional.
- Make sure you only use Natural oils. Scents like: Lavender, Chamomile and Orange have a calming affect. Eucalyptus of course is great for colds and sore throats.

Homeopathy is very popular in Europe and is slowly becoming more so in North America. It is basically non-toxic, easy to administer and does not cause side affects. It comes in tablet, pellet and liquid forms and should be taken without food, especially peppermint, or any other substance in your mouth. Homeopathic remedies stimulate the body's own defense mechanisms in order to conquer the problem. Companies like: Hyland's, Boiron, NatroBio and Standard Homeopathics are gaining popularity.

Remember to see your child as a whole person, with many different needs—emotional needs are just as important as the physical. Love and support build self-esteem and confidence. Remember to give lots of hugs and kisses and teach proper health by example. As being a parent is also a learning process don't expect perfection from yourself, but if you find yourself taking out your anger and frustration on your child, do something about it. There are parent help lines, books, videos, classes and counseling. Just do your best, as it is the hardest job in the world!

PART TWO

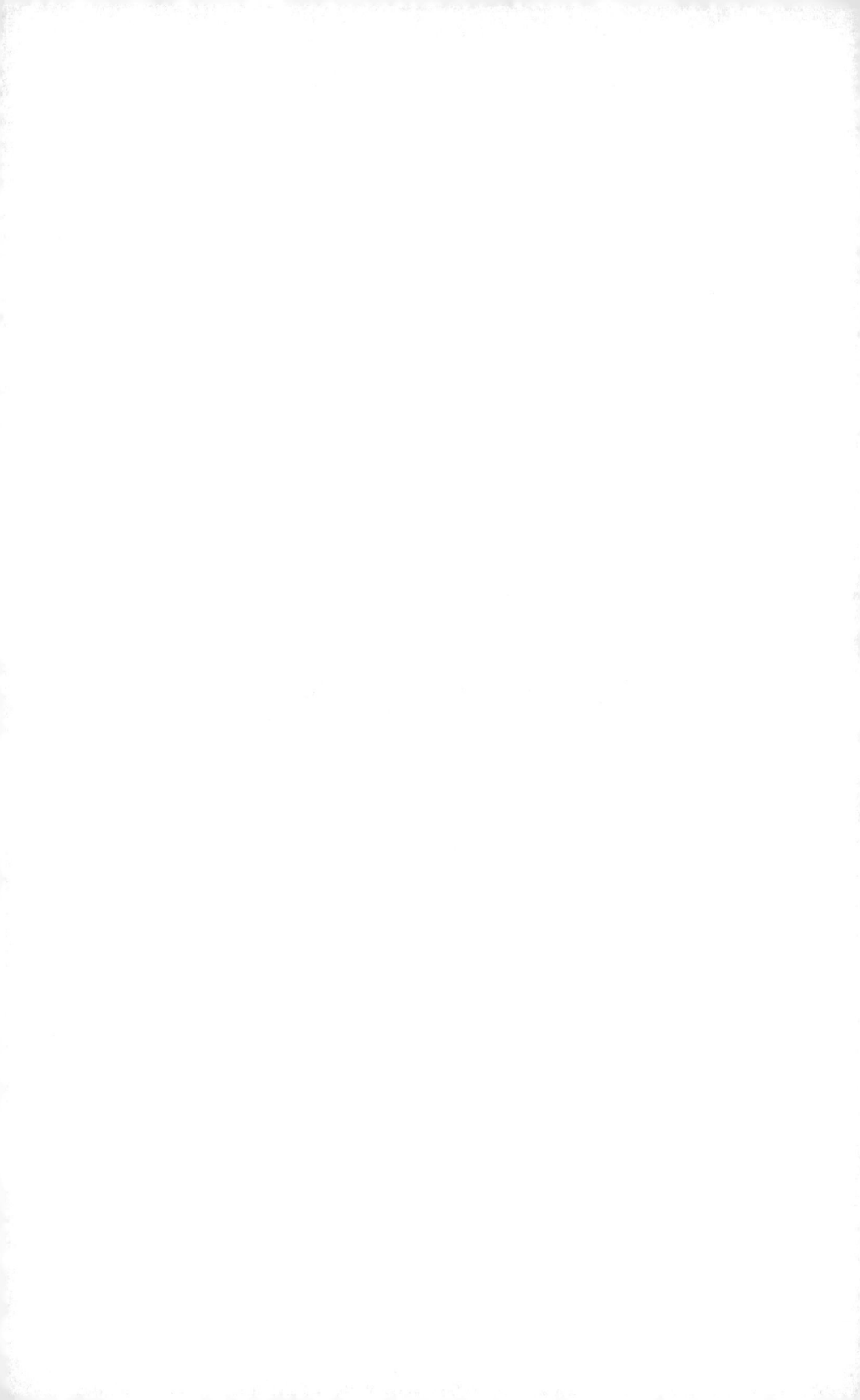

SPECIFIC CONDITIONS AND THEIR REMEDIES

ADD (Attention Deficit Disorder)

First you must look at the diet. Read the labels and take anything with artificial colours, flavours, caffeine, MSG and aspartame out of the diet. Next, get your child tested for allergies, or keep a journal yourself. Observe what he/she craves and eats a lot of. Any food can be the cause, even if it is promoted as healthy. Take your child off of dairy, then wheat, corn, gluten, and chocolate, as these are the most common reactions. Cut back on sugar (candy, cookies, pop, ketchup, etc.) and white flour products, white breads, pastries, cookies and white rice, these turn into sugar in the body. You may mix white and brown rice, if straight brown rice is too much for your child, at least there will be fiber in that combination. Have your child tested for hypoglycemia and diabetes. Many studies have been done on diet and ADD. When a child is taken off the food that triggers the behaviour, he becomes more calm and normal, then the food is introduced and the disruptive behaviour starts again. Remember to take the caffeine (colas), and the artificial colours, especially red, out of the diet first. What we eat and drink influences our health, emotions, mental capability and behaviour more than we realize.

Studies are now being done on the relation between TV watching and ADD; they are finding that TV is affecting ADD.[5]

Supplements to help:

- Essential Fatty Acids (EFAs), fish oils (do not rely on Cod or Halibut liver oils as they will provide too much Vitamins A and D), Evening Primrose Oil, Flax Oil and their combinations. Products such as: Efalax Focus, Focus, Learning Factors, all contain EFAs and are geared towards ADD.
- A good natural multi-vitamin-mineral pill, Nubears, Friends, or any of the other natural companies, taken with breakfast or lunch.
- Vitamin C with Bioflavonoids 500mg to 2000mg, divide the doses if higher than 500mg. Loose bowels will result if too much is taken at once. .
- Calcium & Magnesium, 1000mg or more for an adult, half of this for a child that is half the adult size and again for a smaller child. Buy it in chewable or liquid form and give it in the evening as it helps to calm.
- Zinc, which can be given in lozenge form, 10-15mg a day.

ALLERGIES, HAY-FEVER, SENSITIVITIES

There are many things a body can react too, so this is a much broader subject than can be covered here. Everyone's body is different so even with the help of a good book, or seeking the help of a professional; each person will react differently to the same substance. Keep a Journal.

Chemical Sensitivities are becoming more and more prominent. Our bodies are bombarded with so many chemicals that we become overloaded, causing reactions and sickness to occur. Our children are so much smaller so their bodies are even less able to cope with the many chemicals in our air, food, water, cleaners, beauty products and yard care products. By using natural cleaners, beauty care, deodorizers, lawn care products and consuming pure water and food, you can help your children stay away from too many chemicals. If you suspect there are heavy metals and other chemicals involved in their poor health, then tests like Hair Analysis, Live Blood Cell Testing and others could be done. There are so many natural cleaning products on the market now, along with shampoos, soaps (laundry, dish and bar) and even deodorizers. Think about what you spray in the house and the yard—use natural products as much as you can and on warm days open your windows and air out your house and also your car.

The body becomes overloaded with chemicals, unable to get them out. Conditions can develop such as: behavior problems, allergies, MS symptoms, poor immune functioning and more. If you find your child's body contains chemicals and heavy metals, then seek the help of a professional.

Hay fever is another condition we suffer with. First you have to look at the child's diet and take out the white sugar, white flour and other chemicals. Make sure they get enough pure water and fruits and veggies. There are some great homeopathic remedies on the market for allergies to pollens, grass, dust, trees and even animals. Homeopathics are safe and easy to administer, just remember to give them without food, juice, (especially anything with mint) or brushing their teeth within 15 minutes before and after the doses. Wait longer after using mint gum or toothpaste. Do not store these products on top of or close to microwaves or other electrical appliances. Match the symptoms of the child to the symptoms on the label.

Other supplements to build your child's system to make them less susceptible to airborne allergies:

- Grape seed (might be hard to get into a smaller child)
- Essential Fatty Acids
- Cod/Halibut Liver Oil
  Vitamin C with Bioflavonoids
- Quercetin
- Nettles, give in cooled tea form
- Moducare

Food Allergies and Sensitivities are becoming more and more common with our children. You will find they are genetic, but some children can also have these conditions when their parents don't. As talked about in Chapter Five: keep a journal (what they eat, drink, how they look, feel and the times and days), seek the help of a professional (Naturopathic Dr., etc.) and become educated. Read the labels and take out all artificial colours, flavours, caffeine, MSG, Aspartame and cut back on sugar and white flour products. If the symptoms still exist, then take out dairy and wheat, next, corn, gluten, chocolate and anything else that is a suspect. Often, it is what the child eats a lot of and craves that is the problem. There are so many foods on the market that do not contain dairy, wheat and other allergic foods. You will find them in health stores and natural food sections. To not develop further allergies, use a Rotation Diet—rotate what is eaten on a day-to-day basis.

Supplements to help build their systems:
- Vitamin C with Bioflavonoids
- Calcium Magnesium (liquid and chewable)
- Acidophilus
- Quercetin
- Multi-Vitamin Mineral pill (chewable)
- Digestive Enzymes
- Juice+ Gummies

A further note on allergies, your child may be reacting to the chemicals on the foods, not the foods themselves, so try organic. Dust and molds may also be the problem, so keep the surroundings free from dust and molds, with natural cleaners. Never give them tap water, as it is full of chemicals.

APPETITE, POOR

When your child has a poor appetite, he/she needs more nutrition and you also need to check that there is not something else going on, like stress, depression or some other illness. Cut down on the amount of juice, candy and junk food given. Do not give liquids before or with the meals. Ask your child what healthy foods they would like to eat. Try giving them a protein blender drink, with milk (or Soya milk), greens, flax oil, protein powder, bananas and frozen strawberries, for breakfast. Rebars are also a healthy food, with two cups of fruits and two of vegetables in one bar and it tastes like fruit leather.

Supplements to help increase appetite:
·   Biostrath from Bioforce
·   A natural children's multi-vitamin mineral pill
·   Zinc lozenges (helps with taste)
·   Herbal Tea: catnip, fennel, ginger, peppermint (cooled.)

ASTHMA

If your child has asthma, cut back on sugar and white flour products. Eat more fresh fruits and vegetables, garlic, onions, nuts, seeds, whole grains and brown rice. Drink more pure water and start to include green drinks. You might need to cut out dairy and maybe even wheat if you find they have an allergic reaction to them. Also check to see if there is an allergy to dust, or a reaction to chemicals in the home. Beware of food additives such as: sulphites and artificial colours, which have been known to cause attacks.

Supplements to help:

- Respiractin (they make a children's formula)
- Quercitin
- Vitamin C with Bioflavonoids
- Calcium Magnesium
- EFA's
- A multi-vitamin-mineral pill
- Grape Seed
- Mullein, Slippery Elm, Licorice Root and Golden Seal

Do not give them any formula containing Ephedra.

AUTISM

Feed your child more raw fruits, vegetables, whole grains, brown rice, raw nuts, seeds, beans and other unprocessed foods. Make sure they get enough fiber and good quality proteins (white turkey, chicken, tofu, and protein powders). Cut back on sugars, white flour, caffeine, salt, chocolate, pop, candies, cookies and anything else refined. Check for food allergies. Drink more pure water, exercise and do deep breathing. Eat small meals every few hours to keep a constant supply of energy to the brain. Include EFA's in their diet, either in pill or liquid form.

Supplements:

- Calcium Magnesium, liquid or chewable
- Lecithin Granules
- Gingko Biloba
- Multi-vitamin-mineral pill
- Vitamin C with Bioflavonoids
- Vitamin E (natural source, d-alpha) 400IU for 100+lbs., 200IU/50lbs, etc.
- EFA's, Flax oil, Focus, Salmon Oil, Primrose Oil.

BRAIN (Learning Disabilities)

Read the last section on autism. Be aware that all children develop at their own speed in each area of development. Studies have shown that girls have a larger area in the brain for language and tend to develop language better and faster, using more words than boys. If you are worried about your child in any way, get a good book and see a specialist to determine if there really is a problem.

Supplements to help:

- The supplements suggested for Autism
- Essential Fatty Acid products: Efalex Focus, Focus, Learning Aid, etc.
- A good quality protein powder

BRUISES and SPRAINS

If your child is on a better diet, he will injury himself less and heal faster. Better health leads to more clarity, energy, co-ordination and an over-all good feeling emotionally and physically. When your child does hurt himself, try these remedies:

- Arnica—as an ointment on the bruise or the sprain or the swelling (do not use on broken skin.)
- Arnica—as homeopathic tablets, pellets, or liquid. Take this as soon as possible after the injury and for every two hours until condition improves (use every 15 min. if in a lot of pain). Always take homeopathics in an empty mouth, no food, drink, gum, and toothpaste for 15-30 minutes before and after dose.

Arnica can be used after operations, dental work and broken bones.

CHICKENPOX (Measles, Mumps)

Once again, watch the diet and cut back on the sugar, as sugar weakens the immune system making them more susceptible to everything. Give lots of pure water, fresh natural juices and natural vegetable broths. Catnip tea is calming and good to help with the fever. Giving the homeopathic remedies like: Belladonna, Aconite, Bryonia and others are safer than giving Aspirin. Studies have shown an increased risk of Reye's Syndrome[6] when children are given aspirin to lower a fever; a fever is the body fighting the virus. Just remember to take your child's temperature and if it rises above 103 F, seek medical attention.

Supplements to help:

- Vitamin C with Bioflavonoids— 2000 - 4000 a day divided doses
- Vitamin A—10,000 - 20,000 daily (or for smaller doses give a children's multi-vitamin, or cod liver oil) Do not give this dose after illness is over.
- Beta Carotene—10,000 daily (Remember to half the dose for a child half the size of an adult and give a child still smaller a quarter of the dose.)
- For the skin, use teas like: chamomile, Echinacea, ginger and oatmeal in baths or wet compresses.
- Belladonna is great for a red hot fever.

COLDS COUGHS THE FLU

It is normal for a child to catch some colds, coughs and flues when they are first exposed to them; their immune system needs to be built up. Sometimes the child may continuously catch these viruses. When this happens, you need to look into why and how to build their immune system. There are a few reasons for a weakened immune system and we will discuss some of them here: genetics, improper diet, stress, a spinal subluxation, infrequent bowel movements, toxins or heavy metals in the body, lack of fresh air and exercise, lack of certain vitamins, minerals, EFAs, water and improper hygiene practices.

Genetics can mean we are susceptible to certain kinds of illnesses and conditions. It can also provide us with low levels of important vitamins, minerals, EFAs and other substances. Improper diet and stress can further deplete these substances. Lack of fresh air and exercise will mean the body is not getting enough oxygen into its cells and also the important substances are not getting into the cells, while the toxins will be unable to leave the body. If the body is unable to remove the toxins through the proper channels—the bowel, urine, skin and lungs, it will continue to circulate them and eventually deposit them somewhere. This in turn will clog up the body, causing fatigue, inactivity, and illness.

When a child is born and throughout his/her life, the spine will move out of place causing a lack of nerve energy to a specific organ or area of the body. When this is corrected by a trained chiropractor, the energy can flow freely and help the organs fight against illness.

Heavy Metals and other chemicals can weaken the immune system, which is why we should use natural cleaners, sprays, shampoos, lotions and weed killers. The chemicals used around the home are said to be the most toxic of all. Mercury fillings have also been shown to weaken the immune system. If you suspect your child has heavy metal toxicity then there are tests such as Live Blood Cell and Hair Analysis available.

Once again, diet plays a role in the immune system; sugar and white flour products, (white pasta, white rice, pastries, etc.) all turn into sugar in the body. A little bit of this sugar can put down the immune system for hours afterwards, leaving the door open for any virus you encounter. Corn syrup, honey, fructose, brown sugar and juices (yes, even orange juice), all have the same affect. Drink water, herbal teas and broths instead. Do not substitute Aspartame, thinking it is safer—it is not. Aspartame kills your brain cells and even sets off seizures in some people. Everything discussed here has a greater affect on the smaller body of a child. Eat more fresh fruits and vegetables, whole grains and good quality proteins.

Supplements to help build the immune system and fight the virus:

- Vitamin C with Bioflavonoids (use Ester C if your child is sensitive to regular C)
- Zinc Lozenges
- Cod or Halibut Liver Oil
- Echinacea, or Echinacea/Goldenseal combinations (do not use longer than a week at a time, or during pregnancy)
- Astragalus, Greens + for kids.
- Ginger
- Acidophilus (you may open a capsule and mix it in good quality, natural yogurt.)
- Homeopathic remedies specific to the condition. (Match the symptoms of the child to the symptoms on the box—give in an empty mouth)
- Herbal or Homeopathic Cough Syrups
- Aromatherapy, Eucalyptus in an ointment rubbed on the chest area—do not use on babies or get into eyes.

COLIC

Colic is often due to a food reaction; the first food to suspect is usually dairy. Take yourself, if breastfeeding, and your child off of all dairy. Other foods that can cause reactions are: chocolate, caffeine, wheat, strong spices, strawberries, oranges and bananas. Keep a journal, write down everything you have done and note if there is any improvement, etc. Having the spine adjusted by a trained chiropractor can also help colic.

Natural Remedies for Colic:

- Homeopathic remedies by Hyland's, Boiron and others.
- Cool teas: fennel, catnip, chamomile, and mint.

CONSTIPATION

Constipation should not last more than a couple days. In fact, we should ideally have a bowel movement after every meal and at least every day. Add more pure water, fiber, fruits and vegetables and of course dried fruits (prunes and raisins). Add EFAs to the diet, flax oil, or other oil formulas (Udo's Oil, Essential Balance, etc.) Give them 1 tablespoon for 100 lbs, 1 teaspoon-1/2 tablespoon 50 lbs. Also massaging their feet in the intestinal area, according to the Reflexology chart at the back of the book, can help get things moving again. If constipation persists, see a doctor.

Supplements to help:
- Acidophilus
- Vitamin C 500mg to 2000mg, with Bioflavonoids
- Calcium & Magnesium (liquid or chewable form)—an adult dose is 1000mg a day of Calcium, half that for a child half the size and so on.
- Essential Fatty Acids

CRADLE CAP

With this condition, you also need to check the diet for food reactions with dairy then wheat being the first two to go. Add essential fatty acids to the diet, either to the mother (if breastfeeding), or to the child. Flax oil, Udo's Oil, Essential Balance oil are all great choices. Add 1 tablespoon in a protein drink for the mother, or a quarter teaspoon in baby's food after it is heated or cooked. Never heat or cook these oils, as the heat turns them into a bad fat.

Shampoo baby's hair with a mild natural baby shampoo—check the ingredients to make sure it is natural. Before shampooing, rub a little almond or jojoba oil into the scalp and let it sit for five minutes, then shampoo. After this, comb it out with a fine tooth comb.

CROUP

Feed the child a lot of fluids, pure water, herbal teas and homemade soups. Use Eucalyptus oil in a vaporizer and get them to inhale the steam. Put the oil into a carrier oil (almond or jojoba) and rub into the chest: 1 oz. carrier oil, 2 drops eucalyptus, 1 drop tea tree oil. Rub it on throat and chest 1-2 times a day. Do not use this on babies under 6 months old. Do not get in eyes or in mouth.

Supplements to help:
- Vitamin C—200mg for 6-12 month-olds in divided doses, 300-400 mg for 1-3 yr-olds in divided doses, and 500mg-2000mg over 4 yrs-old in divided does.
- Zinc Lozenges, 5mg a day for 6-12 month olds, 10mg for 1-3 yr olds and 15-20mg for over 3 yrs.
- Cod Liver Oil
- A natural Children's multi-vitamin-mineral pill
- Respiractin Children's formula.

EAR INFECTIONS

Ear infections are 70 % due to a dairy allergy, so take them off of dairy, if the condition continues, get them allergy tested. Build up their immune systems; cut back on the sugars and white flour products. There are natural ear drops that can also be used.

ECZEMA and OTHER SKIN PROBLEMS

With skin problems you need to first check the laundry soaps and the skin products you use with your child. Switch to a natural laundry soap, natural bar soap (Olive Oil is good), natural lotions and shampoos also. The less chemicals used the better, as regular soaps, lotions and shampoos are so full of chemicals, that they overload the body, so the body trys to get rid of them through the skin. Most of the time, you will not find the ingredient listings on the body care products.

Then you look at the diet, to see if there are any food allergies or reactions. Take out the unnatural foods, artificial colours, flavours, msg, aspartame and other chemicals. Your child might have a dairy allergy, so take them off of all dairy for two weeks, to see if the skin clears up. Keeping a food journal is good; record food, drinks and any reactions. The next food to eliminate is wheat, then all gluten; gluten is contained in many grains and is often added to regular foods. You will find there are many gluten-free products available in health food stores and some grocery stores. Corn and chocolate can also cause reactions.

Supplements to help skin conditions:
·   Essential Fatty Acids (good fats), Fish oils, Primrose oil, Flax oil, Hemp oil. You can get a lot of these flavoured for kids now. You can also put this in a protein blender drink.
·   A Natural Children's Multi-vitamin, the B vitamins are good for the skin.
·   Greens + for Kids
·   Vitamin C, natural flavours and colours
·   Natural ointments containing herbs

FATIGUE

Tiredness can be caused by a number of things, so it is good to visit your Doctor. Some causes are: blood sugar problems, diabetes, allergies, not sleeping well enough and low iron levels. After you have had the necessary tests by the Doctor, and you know what is wrong, see the appropriate section in this book. A child has a lot of growing to do, so their iron can be low, give them liquid Iron, Floradix is good, 10mg a day in a little juice; do not give iron with their Calcium supplement. During pregnancy, if the mother did not have enough iron, which is often the case, the child will be born without enough iron, so watch for tiredness, low immune system and inability to recover from sports as your child grows up.

GROWING PAINS

Calcium-Magnesium, given in liquid or chewable forms. Remember to shake the bottle if you get the liquid as the calcium tends to settle to the bottom.

HEADACHES

Headaches can be caused from a few different triggers. If your child has had persistent headaches, take them to a doctor.

Here are some of the causes of headaches:
- allergies to foods and/or chemicals
- a neck subluxation, stress
- an overloaded school backpack
- constipation
- eyestrain
- sinus pressure
- caffeine consumption
- Other causes

Finding the cause and correcting it is the first thing to do.

Your child could be reacting to chemicals in the air (household products) and/or chemicals in foods. Stay away from MSG, aspartame, sulfites, fermented foods (vinegars, cheeses), and also dairy and wheat. Keep a food and symptoms journal to help you determine the causes. If you feel it is a subluxation, see a trained chiropractor. Talk to your child about the stresses and worries of their life and work on resolving them. Recent studies have shown the negative effect on the back and neck from carrying backpacks that are too heavy. Constipation can be a problem if it lasts for days; the toxins re-circulate in the blood stream, which can be the cause of headaches and other problems. Ideally, a bowel movement should happen after every meal—certainly every day. See the section on constipation for what to do. Take your child to a doctor to have her eyes and sinus areas checked if you feel this is where the problem lies. Sinus infections can be caused by chemicals, food allergies, sugars, and a weakened immune system.

Supplements to help:

- Calcium & Magnesium, liquid or chewable form—500mg-1000mg depending on the size/age of the child, give in divided doses.
- Essential Fatty Acids—1 teaspoon-1 tablespoon (50lbs. – 1 tsp., 100 lbs. – 1 Tbsp.)
- B Vitamins (can be found in a good children's multi, also in liquid form)
- Vitamin C with Bioflavonoids—500mg - 2000mg (divided doses if over 500mg)
- Ointments are available to be rubbed on the neck and the temple.
- Try massaging the sore area or the foot according to chart in back of book (digestion, liver, big toe area)

HEAD LICE

Head Lice is quite common once your child goes to school. Once again, make sure your child's diet is good to ensure a strong immune system, so cut back on the sugar! One 12oz. soda has about 9 teaspoons of sugar. White flour products, including regular pasta, also turn into sugar in the body. Supplements like garlic and cod liver oil will also boost their immune systems so they are not so susceptible to lice and other conditions.

If your child does get head lice, Tea Tree Oil is one of the best remedies. Smother them by covering the head with olive oil mixed with a few drops of Tea Tree Oil. Leave this on for a few hours or overnight. Cover the head with a shower cap or towels so you don't get olive oil everywhere. Put 8-10 drops of Tea Tree oil in a Tea Tree Oil shampoo. Lather well and keep it on for 5 minutes. Use this shampoo daily until the threat of lice is gone. Do not get Tea Tree Oil in the eyes.

Remember to comb the hair with a lice comb and pick out every nit. Wash all bedding, clothes and towels—dry in a hot dryer. Put all stuffed animals in the freezer overnight. Put all pillows in a hot dryer for 30 minutes. Vacuum the couch, bed, and floors. Repeat this in 7-10 days. Examine the hair closely on a regular basis until all nits are gone.

INSOMNIA & NIGHTMARES

It is very discouraging when you are so tired, and your child won't go to sleep! First, make sure they are not getting caffeine during the day and especially not in the evening. Do not give them sugar, juice, white flour products, or any refined carbohydrate before bed. Make sure they are not hungry as some children cannot sleep if they are hungry. Feed them: turkey, tuna, yogurt, bananas, figs, milk, soy milk, cheese and nut butters on whole grain bread or crackers, before bed.

Have a nightly bedtime routine and a regular bedtime. Read them a story or two, then let them read a book if they are not tired yet.

Supplements to help:
- Lavender Oil—put a few drops in their bath, put some in a diffuser, or a couple drops on a Kleenex beside their pillow.

- Calcium & Magnesium, liquid or chewable—give it to them with their snack or their dinner. 500mg - 1000mg of calcium with 250mg - 500mg magnesium (give in divided doses with meals throughout the day if giving the higher dose).
- Calm's Forte, Seronol, or other homeopathic remedies
- A natural children's multi with breakfast or lunch
- Cooled Sleepytime Tea

If your child is having nightmares, try these remedies and also talk to them about their dreams to see if there's anything they need. After purchasing a dreamcatcher and hanging it on her bedroom wall, my daughter seemed to have less nightmares. Himalayan Salt Lamps are also useful to better a child's sleep. Prayer can also be used to help ease their nightmares and to combat the monsters!

MEASLES

Seven to fourteen days after initial contact with the measles virus, your child can become ill. Make sure he/she gets more rest, avoids sugary, processed foods and drinks a lot of fluids, including soup broths and cooled herbal teas. Keep the lights dim, so their eyes won't hurt. Watch for other conditions after the measles have gone: ear infections, bronchitis, strep throat, croup and pneumonia. Work on boosting their immune through diet and supplements if this happens.

Supplements to help:
- Cod Liver Oil
- Vitamin C with Bioflavonoids—1000 - 3000mg in divided doses
- Zinc Lozenges—1 - 3 10mg lozenge(s) a day.
- A natural children's multi (for the B vitamins), or liquid B's.

MENINGITIS

Meningitis can progress very quickly, so if you suspect it, take your child to the hospital right away. The infection may seem like a cold or flu, so also look for these signs:

· a red/purple skin rash
· stiff neck
· delirium
· vomiting
· headache
· irritability
· loss of appetite
· a high fever
· respiratory problems
· sensitivity to light
· poor muscle tone.

In babies, specifically, also look for: a bulging soft spot (fontanel) and a high-pitched cry. When the risk of death and serious problems are over and the child is sent home, there are things you can do to help him/her recover and strengthen their immune system. Make sure they get lots of rest in a dimly lit room. Feed him/her lots of natural fluids, along with fruits, veggies, raw nuts, natural yogurts and whole grains. Avoid processed foods.

Supplements to help:

· Acidophilus—there are children's formulas available.
· Vitamin C—1000 - 3000mg in divided doses.
· Zinc Lozenges—1-3 10mg lozenges a day.
· Cod liver Oil
· Echinacea and Goldenseal (do not take longer than a week and do not take during pregnancy)

STREP THROAT

Give your child a healthier diet, with no sugar and lots of fluids. Use all the immune booster Supplements, Vitamin C, Echinacea and other Children's herbal formulas. Zinc Lozenges are good to suck on, if the child is old enough for this. Give them a 10-15mg lozenge three times a day.

SUNBURN

Protect against sunburn—wear hats, drink lots of water, keep a long-sleeved shirt handy and use your natural sunscreen! It is good to get some sun, but just use your common sense and do everything in moderation. To find out how long you should stay in the sun, take your sunscreen strength, multiply it by the time it takes you to burn (SPF 30 x 15 minutes = 450 minutes (7 hours, 50 minutes). Do not stay out longer than this and remember to re-apply sunscreen after swimming and showering. It is important to wear a hat and drinks lots of water (not pop), as heat stroke can still occur. Children are often warm to begin with, so watch them more carefully. Prevention is better than sunburn.

In order to absorb Vitamin D from the sun, you need to have exposed skin in the sun for 10-15 minutes and then do not shower for half an hour to allow the absorption of the vitamin.

If sunburn does occur, here are some natural remedies:
- Aloe Vera Gel
- Vitamin E oil and vitamin E internally
- Vitamin C topically and internally
- Chamomile tea and Rosehip tea—use the cooled tea bags to place over the burn, as long as it is not an open wound.

- A salve made out of herbs like: Calendula, St. John's Wort, Comfrey and Tea Tree Oil (full strength Tea Tree Oil might sting too much.)
- A bath of: Chamomile Flowers, Lavender Oil (a few drops) or Oatmeal will help to soothe the burn.
- *If the sunburn is severe, go to the hospital.*
- Take other Antioxidants such as: CoQ10, Beta Carotene and Zinc—this will help with the healing.
- Eat lots of fresh fruits and Vegetables, for the water and phyto-nutrient content.
- Take Essential Fatty Acids (good fats) and eat good quality proteins.
- Take a natural multi-vitamin-mineral pill.
- L-Glutamine is good for immune function and healing after a burn—add a teaspoon to applesauce for your child everyday. (Do not give if the child had Reye's Syndrome, liver disease or renal failure.)

TEETH GRINDING

Eat more fiber, with vegetables, whole grains, fruits, nuts and other good quality proteins. Eat small meals every 3-4 hours to avoid low blood sugar. Before bed only eat a high protein snack—no sugars, including white flour products and juices, a few hours before bed.

Supplements to help:

- Calcium and Magnesium—500mg - 1000mg, depending on the age/weight of the child and give in divided doses. Buy in chewable or liquid form. 1000mg for 100lbs., 500mg for 50lbs., etc.
- A good natural children's multi-vitamin-mineral pill, given with breakfast or lunch
- Vitamin C 500mg to 1000mg daily in divided doses.

TEETHING

For teething there are homeopathic remedies that can often help calm the baby, so everyone can sleep. Companies like Hyland's, Boiron, and others make specific teething formulas. You can also give the remedy Chamomilla, if the child is very irritable, Belladonna, if the child is more feverish. These can be given in liquid form, tiny pellets, or tablets that dissolve in a little water. For acute conditions, give every 15-30 minutes, then every few hours after that. Do not give with food, as homeopathics work better in an empty mouth. Homeopathy is safe, with a high rate of success.

TONSILLITIS

First we need to look at the diet and cut back on refined foods, especially sugary, white flour type foods. Check for reactions to foods, especially dairy and wheat. Make sure there are adequate vegetables, fruits and proteins in the diet. Add the good fats to the diet and cut back on the fried, hydrogenated fats. Soda pop and even excessive fruit juices (more than one a day) will lower the immune system, so stay away from them. Remember to drink enough pure water.

Supplements to help:
- Zinc lozenges—5-10mg lozenge up to 4 times daily (only take this many when fighting a virus)
- Vitamin C—500mg every 2 hours until loose bowels are experienced
- Acidophilus—take as directed on the bottle
- Cod Liver Oil
- Herbs like Echinacea and Goldenseal—use these two herbs only when needed, not on a continuing basis (do not use goldenseal if pregnant). Also use other herbal formulas designed for boosting the child's immune system.

- Cooled Catnip tea or the homeopathic remedy Belladonna can be given for the fever.

TOOTH DECAY

The first thing you must teach your child is to brush their teeth on a regular basis. Be sure to take them to the dentist for their check-ups and cleaning. Once again, the diet plays a large role in your children's teeth. If he/she eats lots of sugar and refined carbohydrates, there is a greater chance for tooth decay. Stay away from soda pop, it promotes the loss of tooth enamel. Raw vegetables and fruits, like apples, actually have a cleansing affect on the teeth. If your child does eat sweets and sticky, refined foods, then be sure to get them to brush their teeth afterwards.

Supplements to help:
- Calcium and Magnesium, chewable or liquid form
- An adult dose is 1000mg of calcium a day, 500mg of magnesium, give in divided doses. Remember to half the adult dose for a child one-half adult size and quarter the dose for a child a quarter the adult size.
- Acidophilus—try to get a children's formula, use as directed on the bottle.
- A natural children's multi-vitamin-mineral pill
- Vitamin D, Cod or Halibut Liver Oil is a good source.

THRUSH

Thrush is Candida, which affects the mouth and sometimes the baby's bottom as a diaper rash. Candida is often due to food allergies, so mother and baby need to look at their diet. Avoid sugars, white flour (pasta, cakes, cookies, etc.), syrups, fermented foods, pickles, chocolate, yeast, mushrooms, aged cheeses, gluten and vinegars. Avoid any other substance you feel either your baby or you might be reacting too. Keep a food/symptom journal as you need to. Cut back on your fruit consumption. Eat more vegetables, brown rice, millet, fish, live culture yogurts and fibers. Use natural cleaners and detergents—all other chemicals used in and around the house should be natural. Buy only cotton underwear and watch for baby's reaction to disposable diapers.

Supplements to help:
- Acidophilus—take as directed either through the mother (if breast feeding), or in a little yogurt for the child/baby (get a children's formula.)
- Multi-vitamin-mineral pill or liquid for baby
- Garlic—as directed on bottle for breast-feeding mother
- Vitamin C—1000mg 3 times a day for mother. For baby, liquid baby vitamins, according to the directions on the bottle.
- Essential Fatty Acids—1 tablespoon daily for mother, half teaspoon daily for baby in milk

VACCINATIONS

Vaccinations are a personal choice. Before you decide, read all you can and learn about the pros and cons. Many children have experienced reactions to the vaccines, some irreversible. Remember, if your child does develop a reaction to the vaccine, DO NOT give any more, The diet talked about for the immune system and the vitamins and herbs can all help to build your child's immune system and thereby make him/her stronger so he/she doesn't catch as many of the vaccinated conditions, Cutting back on sugar is a great help to the immune system. There are homeopathic remedies to help with many conditions and also remedies to help with reactions to the vaccines. Consult a homeopathic doctor for a more personal vaccine replacement for your child, if your child reacts, or if you so desire.

FOOT REFLEXOLOGY

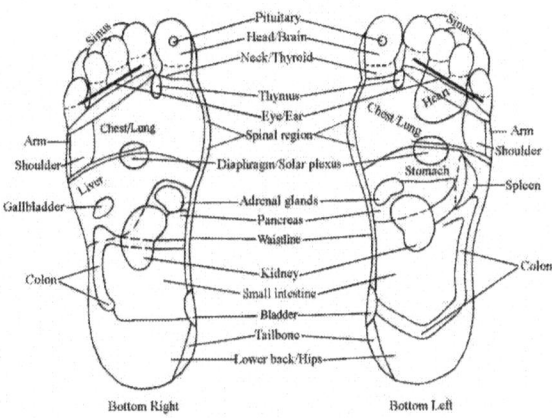

MORE BOOKS ON CHILDREN'S HEALTH

- *"A Pathway to Success"*; Lawrence Weathers, Ph.D.

- *"ADD Nutrition Solution, A Drug Free 30-Day Plan"*; Marcia Zimmerman, Owl Books.

- **"ADD/ADHD",** Dr. E. Ali ND.

- **"ADHD Alternatives",** Aviva Romm, CPM., AHG, Tracy Romm, ed. D.

- **"Healing Children's Attention and Behavior Disorders",** Dr. Abram hoffer, MD.

- **"Ritalin-Free Kids"**, Judyth Reichenberg-Ullman, ND., Robert Ullman, ND.

- *"Rage Free Kids, Homeopathic Medicine for Defiant, Aggressive and Violent Children"*; Judith Reichenburg Ulman & Robert Ulman.

- *"Children with Starving Brains, a Medical Treatment Guide for Autism Spectrum Disorder"*; Jacquelyn McCandles M.D.

- **"Is Your Child's Brain Starving?"**, Dr. Michael R. Lyon, MD.

- *"Facing Autism"*; Lynn M. Hamilton.

- *"Vaccines, Autism and Childhood Disorders"*; Neil Z. Miller.

- *"Babies with Down Syndrome"*; edited by Karen Stray-Gundersen.

- **"Chemical-Free Kids, How to Safeguard your Child's Diet and Environment"**, Allan Magaziner, D.O., Linda Bonvie and Anthony Zolezzi.

- *"Non-Toxic Baby, Reducing Harmful Chemicals"*; Nancy Green.

- *"Raising Your Spirited Child"*; Mary Sheedy Kurcinka.

- *"Smart Medicine for a Healthier Child"*; Janet Zand, M.D.

- *"How to Raise a Healthy Child in Spite of Your Doctor"*; Robert Mendelsohn, M.D.

- *"No More Antibiotics"*; Mary Ann Block, M.D.

- *"The Complete Kid's Allergy and Asthma Guide"*; Hospital for Sick Children; Dr. Milton Gold.

- *"Super Healthy Kids, Strengthening Your Child's Resistance to Disease"*; Jane Sheppard.

- *"Super Immunity for Kids, What to Feed Your Children"*; Leo Galland, M.D.

- *"Healthy Childhood, Ear Infections"*; Michael Schmidt.

- *"Encyclopedia of Natural Healing for Children and Infants"*; Mary Bove, N.D.

- *"Parents Guide to Food Allergies"*; Marianne Barber.

- *"Homeopathic Medicines for Pregnancy and Childbirth"*; Richard Moskowitz, M.D.

- *"Homeopathy for Children"*; Gabrielle Pinto and Murray Feldman.

- **"Homeopathic Medicine For Children and Infants",** Dana Ullman, MPH.

- *"Vegetarian Children"*; Sharon Yntema.

- *"The Kid Friendly Food Allergy Cookbook"*; Leslie Hammond and Lynne Marie Rominyer.

- *"Cooking with Herb, the Vegetarian Dragon, a Cookbook for Kids"*; Jules Bass.

- *"Hot to Live with a Nut Allergy"*; Chad K, O.H., M.D.

- **"Natural Baby Care"**, Colleen K. Dodt

- *"Yoga for Children with Autism Spectrum Disorders"*; Louise Goldberg.

- *"Yoga for You and Your Child"*; Mark Singleton.

- *"Baby Om, Yoga for Mothers and Babies"*; Lara Staton and Sarah Perron.

BIBLIOGRAPHY

- "Dr. Mercola" at www.mercola.com
    #1 "Cow's Milk, Diabetes Correction Bolstered."
    #2 & #3 "Worrying About Milk."
    #4 "Child Emotional Care Influences Genetic Expression."
    #5 "How Much TV Does Your Child Watch?"
    #6 "Fever In Children, A Blessing In Disguise."
- "Alive" Magazines
- "Prescription for Nutritional Healing",   James F. Balch, MD., Phyllis A. Balch, CNC.

www.ingramcontent.com/pod-product-compliance
Lightning Source LLC
Chambersburg PA
CBHW021244280526
45784CB00005B/2225